A Survivalist's Guide to Surviving

Against the Odds

Shannon Rizzotto

Prepping and Survival Book Series

Mendon Cottage Books

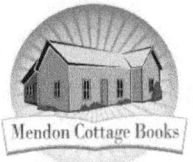

JD-Biz Publishing

All Rights Reserved

Disclaimer

The information in this book is provided for informational purposes only and it is not intended for use as a substitute for proper financial or legal direction by a qualified financial or legal advisor. The information is believed to be accurate as presented based on research by the author.

The author or publisher is not responsible for financial loss or damage incurred by implementing ideas mentioned in this book. The author or publisher is not responsible for errors or omissions that may exist.

Warning

The Book is for informational purposes only and before starting or running any activity or business, it is recommended that you consult with your financial or legal professional. Always follow all laws and regulations mentioned in this book regarding activities, taxes, selling, buying, or ecommerce.

Check out some of the other Entrepreneur Series books
Entrepreneur Series books on Amazon
Check out some of the Science of Living Series books
Science of Living Series on Amazon
Check out some of the Health Learning Series books
Health Learning Series on Amazon

Table of Contents

Introduction

There are times that we may find ourselves in situations where knowing how to survive against all the odds is the one sure thing that WILL in fact save our lives. This book will take you the reader through various scenarios and will show you the basic steps of what you will need in order to survive even the most catastrophic of events.

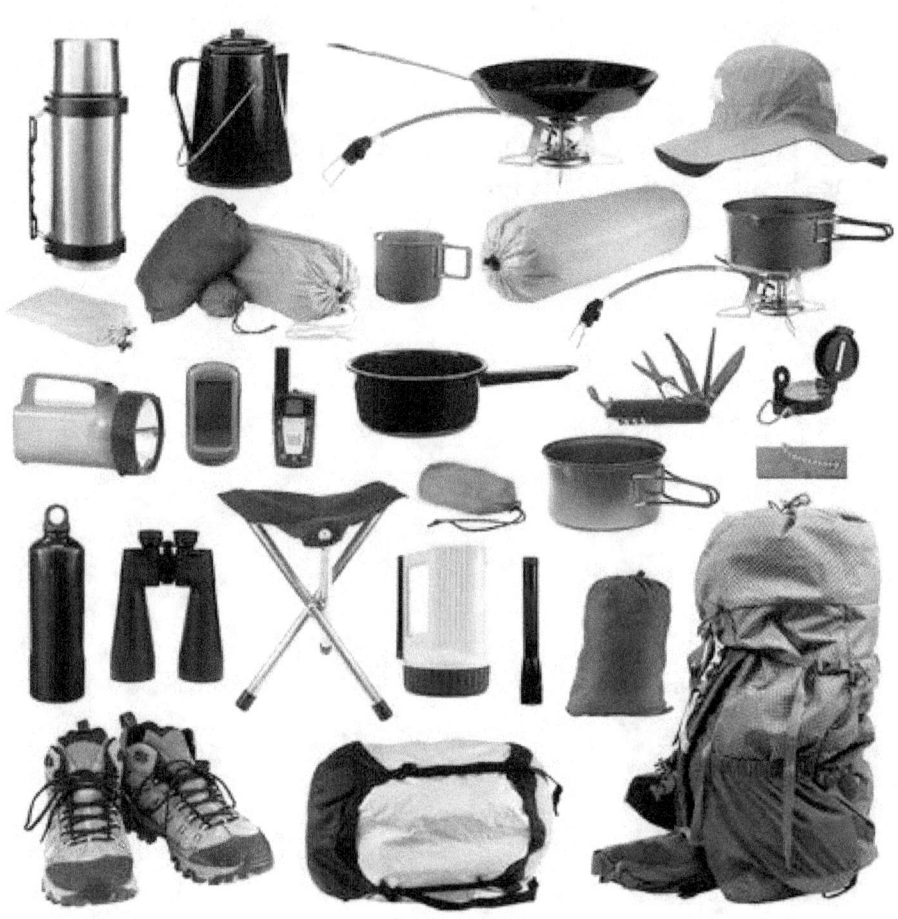

Chapter One - Be prepared

In this day and age even with all of the technology to warn us of disaster it is important to always be ready if it strikes with or without notice. There are several things you will need to do in order to be prepared for any emergency situation. Here is a list of things you will need to be prepared if disaster strikes.

1. A full tank of gas

In any disaster situation having a full tank of gas or access to gas is a dire emergency and can mean the difference between life and death in some cases. Being able to travel to get help, food, water, and even medical treatment will enable you to be one step up on any disaster. Chances are in an extreme situation gas stations will not have power to sell gas or if there is power there is a good chance the nearest gas station will be flooded with customers trying to get out of the area affected by the disaster. So having gas on hand for your vehicle in number one.

2. Water

Regardless what the disaster situation brings you are going to need water. Water is essential in survival. The human body can live without water for just under a week and some have lived a bit longer but this is certainly NOT something you want to either try or risk. You should store at least one gallon of water per person per day for any disaster or survival situation and having up to three weeks' worth of clean drinking water is not out of the question. The human body requires water to survive the amount however, depends on the body type and size of the person. It is said that in a hot environment you need close to a gallon of water per day and children and pregnant or nursing mother's need even more. Have water ready. You will thank yourself in the long run.

3. Food

Food is another necessity and it is important that you have it when needed. The more you do the more calories you burn and, the more calories you burn the more tired you will become so it is important to have plenty of food to keep your body functioning the way you need it to. The human body is capable of going 30 - 40 days without food however, this also depends on the person and the amount of work/movement the person does during the course of the day. In being prepared for any disaster situation have on hand 20-25 cans of both fruit and vegetables. These items can last you a very long time years in fact but in a pinch they will help you maintain the calorie intake you need to survive. If you are in a area where you can hunt or trap live food this is certainly something you can do but, if you are not in an area that affords you this ability it is also a good idea to have protein on hand be it in the form of legumes or canned meat. You can use most canned meats but the very best is Salmon. Salmon meat contains much needed oils and fats required for survival. So, having 10-15 cans in your survival kit would go a long way. Other canned meats to include, tuna fish, chicken, and beef. Some might say ham is a good option but ham contains a lot of salt/sodium and salt causes you to get thirsty. So, if at all possible exclude ham from your stock piled food. If you have shelter after your disaster you may also want to have 10 pounds of the following; flour, pinto beans (dried), rice (white rice has a better shelf life than brown however, you can choose either), chocolate (this can be used as a pick me up when fatigue strikes), sugar and also salt. You can use the salt to cure any live meat you get along the way if needed. Though these foods are pretty basic they will also help you survive.

4. Vitamins

Though certainly needed by the body adding vitamins to your survival kit is not needed but it will certainly add to your survival based on all that your body could potentially be lacking. Multi-vitamins are always a great thing to have on hand and can be bought fairly cheap and contain much of what the body needs on a day to day basis to stay normal.

5. Medicinal Items

(Any suggestions in this section are merely suggestions and should ONLY be considered by a qualified medical advisor. The author's, and/or publisher of this book can not be held responsible for any situation involving misuse of any medications. The author and publisher of this book are not doctors. Use of this information is solely the responsibility of the reader.)

In any survival situation you will want to have various medicinal items available in case your disaster turns into an emergency. Often people overlook their normal prescription drugs the ones they take on a day to day basis that keeps them normal. It is always a smart idea to keep these items handy or easily accessible during any situation. Ibuprophen and Aspirin are great to have on hand as well for fever and minor pain related to any injury sustained during an emergency situation. A first aid kit is always a good thing to have ready for use and should include the following: 2 absorbent compress dressings (5 x 9 inches), 25 adhesive bandages (assorted sizes), 1 adhesive cloth tape (10 yards x 1 inch), 5 antibiotic ointment packets (approximately 1 gram), 5 antiseptic wipe packets2 packets of aspirin (81 mg each), 1 blanket (space blanket), 1 breathing barrier (with one-way valve), 1 instant cold compress2 pair of non-latex gloves (size: large), 2 hydrocortisone ointment packets (approximately 1 gram each), Scissors1 roller bandage (3 inches wide), 1 roller bandage (4 inches wide), 5 sterile gauze pads (3 x 3 inches), 5 sterile gauze pads (4 x 4 inches), Oral thermometer (non-mercury/non-glass), 2 triangular bandages, and tweezers.

Though this is a very basic kit it does include most anything you could need for small issues. For larger issues you will want to seek out medical attention any way you can. (This is where the tank of gas comes in handy.)

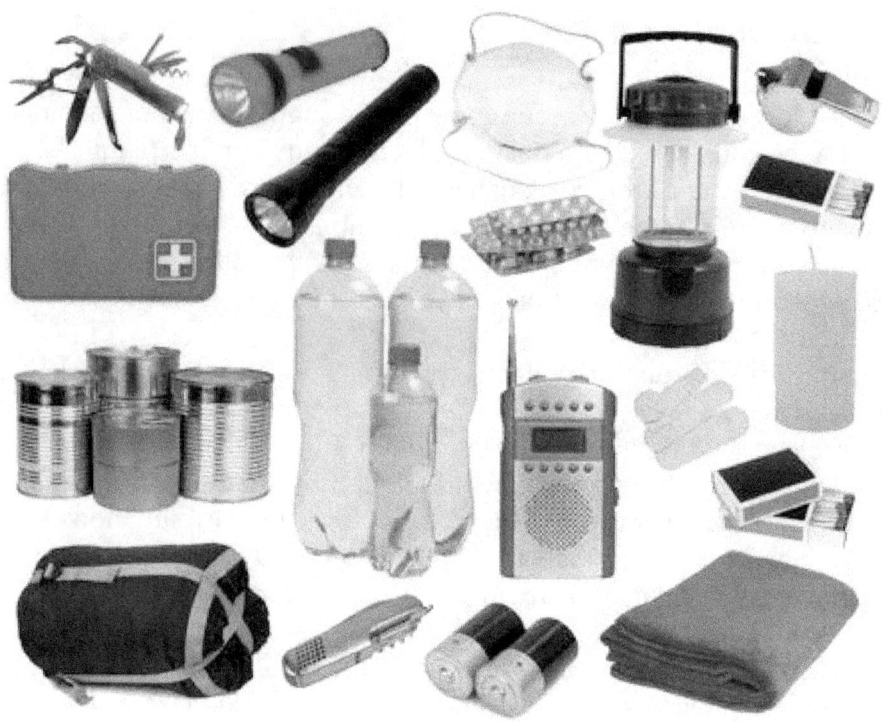

6. Survival Tools

Having certain tools ready for survival and disaster situations is a must and these items include:
A knife, rope, duct tape, waterproof matches, small magnifying glass, 3-4 lighters, sparklers, small folding shovel, blankets, cook-ware, forks/spoons, waterproof bags, and a large candle.

You might not think that some of these items would be any good in a survival situation however, here are some of their uses. Having a good handy knife will be your bread and butter if you will. Without a good knife you will not be able to cut or even craft various items along the way. Duct tape in this day and age is a must have. A good sized industrial roll should be enough. It can be used to make any number of items along the way with a little creativity there is almost nothing you cannot do with duct tape. You can use the waterproof matches, lighters, and even the magnifying glass to start a fire when needed.

Note: (The magnifying glass can only be used on sun filled days). If you cannot find waterproof matches you can make your own with wood stick matches coated in a thin layer of candle wax. This ensures moisture stays away from the sulfur tip and you can light them when needed.

As for the sparklers, you might be thinking, what good will these do? Well, the answer is quite simple. Sparklers burn at temperatures between 1800 - 3000 degrees Fahrenheit so, the use of these as fire starters could be greatly useful. Keep them away from moisture as to ensure their lighting abilities. As for the small folding shovel. You can pick one of these up very around $10.00 and they are great for digging fire pits, base holes for shelters and the list goes on and on. The candle can be used in small quarters at night for minimal light however; it can also be used to waterproof almost anything. Either by melting or by direct pressure rub you can apply wax to any item/s needed.

These are just a few of the basic items you will need for survival. For extended wilderness survival please refer to our other reading material under the survival theme for direct and more focused information on how to survive in any disaster.

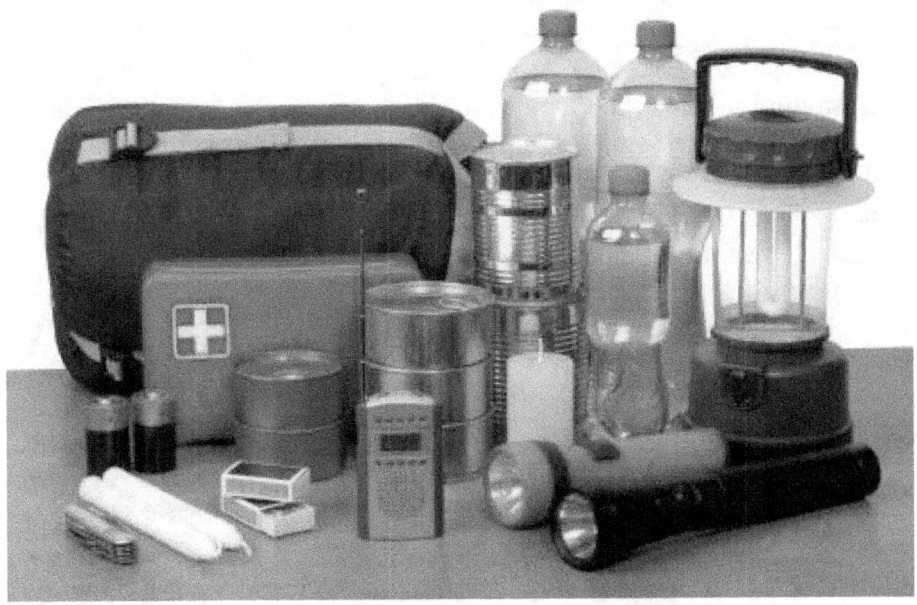

Chapter Two - Surviving the Psychological

(Aspects of a disaster on the mind)

Any disaster situation will wreak havoc on the mind. It is important to stay above it if at all possible. Granted times will certainly be tough and depending on the severity or even the isolation of the disaster event you are going to want to try and stay focused on getting away/out of the situation you find yourself in. We as humans are survivalists by nature but it is easy for doubt to come into play as we find ourselves facing an uncertain future. In any survival situation it will be the small things that will help to put your mind at rest. Like a cup of warm coffee or the heat from a fire you just built. Try taking moments for small victories that will lead to a great mental outcome.

Also, realize that in this day and age the chances of you being rescued are much greater than they were in years past and usually within 24 hours you being searched for. Having a plan will also help you in working towards a goal when faced with the mental aspects of your situation. Setting the overall goal of getting out of your situation is great but, smaller goals are needed to help keep you in the right direction. Building your first fire, building a shelter, etc. these are great smaller goals to keep your mind in a forward progression. The second aspect of the survival situation in the mind is overcoming fear.

Fear is a natural emotion but it is also an emotion we all can control. When fear sets in you need to look at it from all the aspects and sides you are presented with. Try to imagine fear as just a very small piece of the bigger puzzle of surviving and you will be able to overcome it. Sure, any situation where we are forced to find food and shelter can cause fear but taking pleasure in those smaller victories that we talked about a bit ago will work wonders in helping you put fear at bay. The other side to fear is risk. Risk will come with any situation and you want to use your education to take each risk that comes your way.

Example, you are in the wilderness and you are faced with having to cross a ravine. The bad thought process of this situation would be risking your life to climb down into this ravine and then climbing out of it to the other side. An educational risk would have you find a suitable area that is less dangerous and to try to build a crossing to assure you are not putting yourself in harm's way. This said, never take a risk without having a plan to set in motion to counter any negativities of the risk. The other absolutes you need to be aware of are failure and uncertainty. The latter of these two will come with any situation and there is no cure for uncertainty. However, being ready in any given situation is what will set you above the rest. Now when it comes to failure, you will be faced with this often and if fact even in a situation that does not involve survival you are faced with failure however, you fight through it and overcome. This applies in a survival mode as well. Failure can only affect you if you allow it to. There will surely be certain times where it might feel like you are going to fail but, you must think positive and stay focused. In a survival mode failure is not an option and you must never allow it to become one. In order to keep the mind at ease the body needs to stay active. Doing 15 -20 minutes of activity other than what you would be doing in a survival situation will help keep your mind active and you body relaxed. Walking is a great idea plus it gives you the ability to look over your surroundings and survey the landscape for possible help or even a way out.

You will have a better chance of making it through this ordeal if you can get your mind in the right spot. It may not be easy given your situation but keeping a healthy and active mind will aid you in your overall survival.

Chapter Three - How to build a shelter

To build a shelter you will need a few of the tools from the kit I spoke of a few pages ago. The main tools you will use are, the knife, shovel, rope, and duct tape. Here is what you will need to do. First, find a suitable area away from but close to water if at all possible. Higher ground is recommended however, any space clear of rocks, and debris is fine. Clear an area about 5 foot by 5 foot in diameter. This will be your base area for you shelter and camp. If you are in a wooded area find downed tree branches about 2-3 inches in diameter. If you are in a urban area look for any wood or metal debris you can use for your skeleton or the ribs of your structure you are about to build. You will need at least eight of these items. Once you have found either the branches or the metal or wood you will want them to be about 6 feet in length. Place each piece in the four corners of the area you cleared, you can also place the other four in-between each of the four you already have laid out. Now, you want to dig angled holes about 2 feet deep to place one end of each piece into. Two feet deep should be enough to secure each piece to withstand significant wind and provide stability for your structure. Once you have the holes dug you are going to start by placing the pieces you cut into each of the four corners of the shelter base area. You will be using each piece to rest against the other. This should start to look like the frame of a teepee. Once you have the first four set up you will want to secure them together at the top with your rope or you can craft rope from the roll of duct tape however you might want to save the duct tape for rope making later down the road. Once you have the top of the pieces secure, you can now place the other pieces that are in-between your original four pieces in their holes and attach them with more rope to the rest of the structure. Now after you have done this you can start to find the guts of your structure. You can use downed pine, or any other branches you can locate or in a urban area you can use broken wood, siding, really anything you can locate. The idea is to use these to fill in the slots between your frame you just built. You want to weave these between the main polls if at all possible and you can use as much of this as you need however, keep in mind the weight you are putting on the structure and always be safe about how much you use. You will also want to make sure you have an opening in your structure so you can get in and out. Also, keep in mind it is very important to never use fire in your structure as you do not want to burn yourself or it down. Keep fire well away from your structure. Below is an example of how your structure could look.

Now, once you have a basic structure built you will want to make a floor inside. Often people try to build the floor and build around it but, if you build the structure and then add the floor you might find it easier to do and you will know for certain how much space you have to cover with your new floor. To build a floor you can either elevate it or simply pad it. Padding is good and easy IF you are in a well-drained area or if you have limited amounts of building material. To make an elevated floor simply cut branches to fit the inner circumference within your shelter.

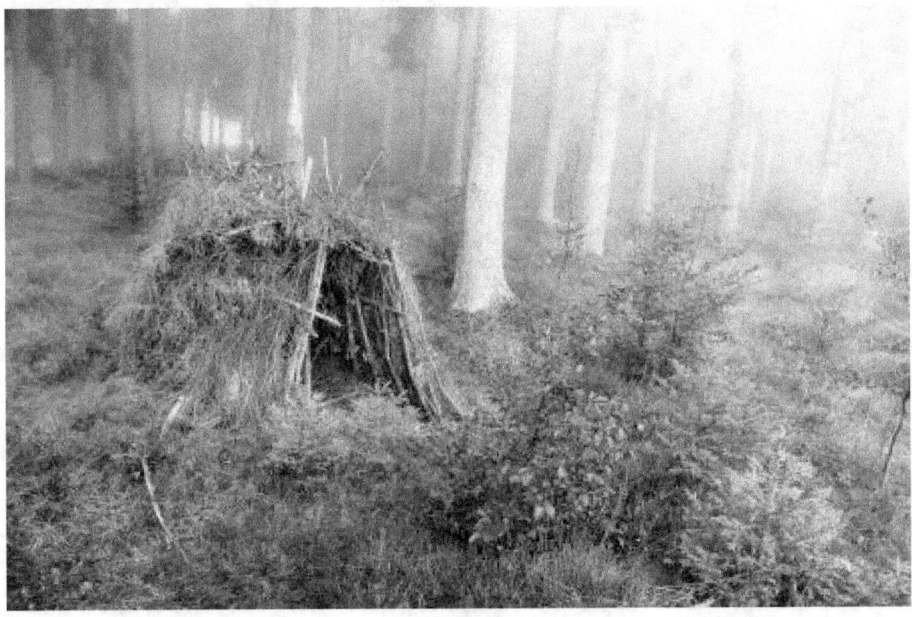

You will want as many as you can fit in the structure and you will want to fit them together as snug as possible. This is where making some rope out of duct tape may come in handy. To make the rope simply fold over the tap so the two sticky ends meet. This should make 1 inch strips. You can then cut these into thinner strips if needed or use them as they are. Take the duct tape rope and tie the flooring together so they do not slide or move when in use. Once the elevated floor is built you can then add a blanket or even soft white pine needles for padding. This will help keep you comfortable and it will also make your shelter smell good. This again can relax not only the body but the mind as well.

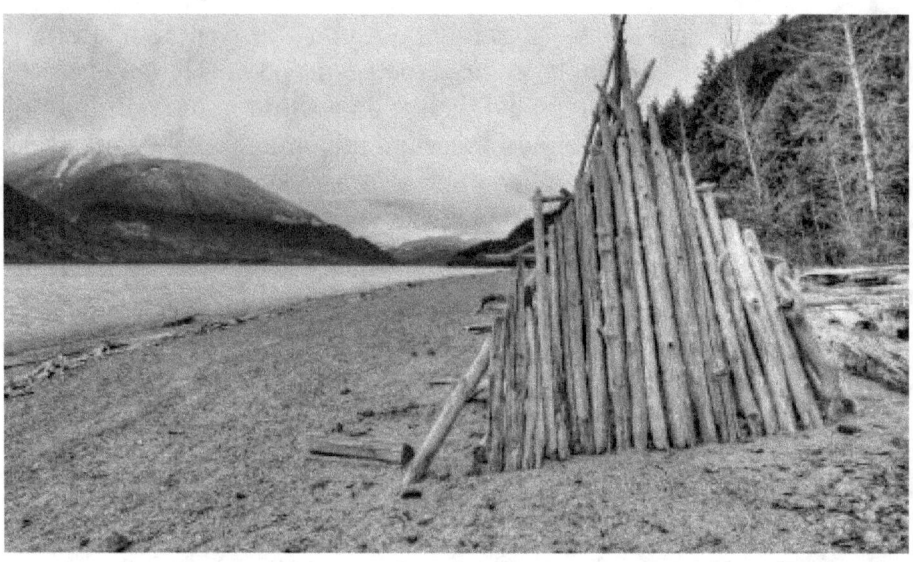

Now, once you have your living shelter constructed there are other structures you may want to construct. A toilet, cooler, storage, dryer, and fire pit. The easiest of these will be your fire pit. To build this you need your shovel and some softball sized rocks if you can find some. Depending on the size of the area you want for your fire pit will determine the size of the hole dug. For a basic fire pit it should be about three feet wide all around. It should also be dug about 6-8 inches deep. Once the pit is dug you can add rocks to the outer edge. Also, you want to make sure when you have a fire lit that no rocks fall into the fire and remain in the fire pit. This can cause the rocks to crack and explode. The moisture in the rocks will become heated and with no place to go it can blow up.

To build a toilet, you want this area well away from your camp area, and your food/drinking water supply. Find an area that is flat and downwind from your camp. You can dig a hole a foot or so deep even deeper if you want. Keep the dirt you dig from the hole on the side of the hole. You will use this to cover up any fecal matter and to keep bugs and flies away. Once the hole is dug, you can fins a few broken logs or branches and set them on the hole to use as a toilet. Make sure to keep the "debris" covered once you are done using this area. You can make many of these as they fill up as needed. Your new toilet pit should look something like the photo below.

Note: you can design or build this structure however you like but the way I described is the easiest.

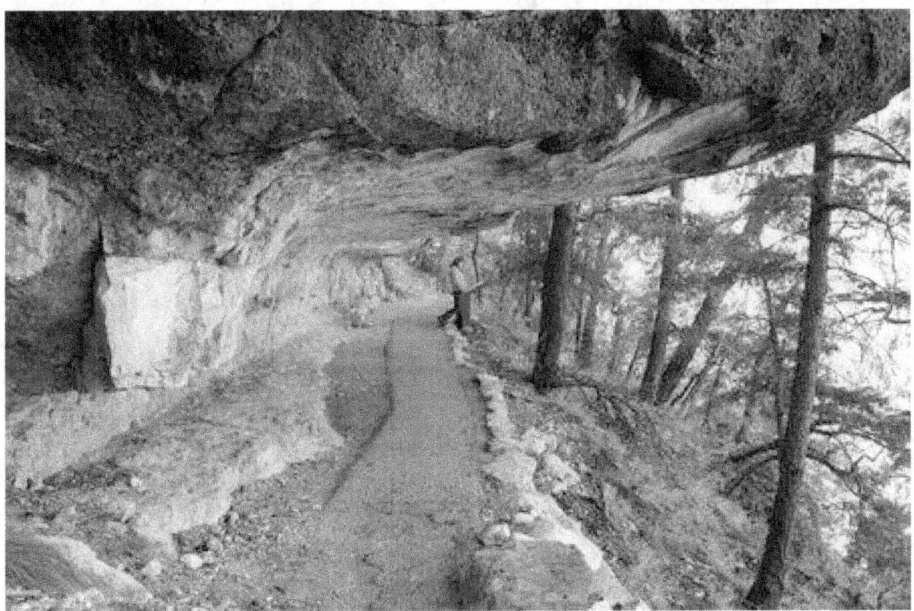

To build a dryer you will need five, six foot poles. These should be 2-3 inches in diameter. You will dig four holes about two feet deep and four feet across. Place each pole in each hole. Make sure you angle the holes so that the poles can lean on each other at which point you will tie two at a time together at the tops. Once you have these poles evenly spaced you will use the fifth pole to connect the four you have tied together at the top running length wise from the first two to the second two. Now tie the fifth pole to the other four and you will have a dryer/drying rack. Basically, and though smaller your new structure should look like the photo below.

Once you have this structure built you can use it for any number of things including: Drying food, cloths, herbs, blankets and even stretching and cleaning hides in an extended type survival scenario.

A drying rack can be used even as a smoker if you dig a fire pit under the rack or place the rack over your existing pit to be used to smoke meats. Be careful that you do not make your fire to large or it could burn the rack making it useless.

Building a storage unit is best done either in the ground close to your base camp or, hanging in the air from a tree. To build one in the ground simply dig a pit a couple of feet deep. Line the bottom with rocks and keep the top covered. You can place items inside this pit to keep them out of the sun and away from the elements. It will also keep them cool. Not cold but cool enough to keep certain items fresh. Now if you want to build a device to hang in a tree, which is good to keep critters away. You can use a bucket, pre-made box or you can use your duct tape to build a bag to hang up high enough to keep would be scavengers from finding your perishable food items.

If you use this method you will want it to be at least two-hundred feet away from your camping area to keep you safe from animals that may try to get to your storage device. As described in the photo below. It is best to make your tree storage device at least twelve feet in the air and six feet off the branch of the tree you are using.

It is very important to NOT draw attention to your camp area and using this type of storage device will help you in many ways. You can use either regular rope or 550 Para cord. You can also make rope out of the duct tape as mentioned before.

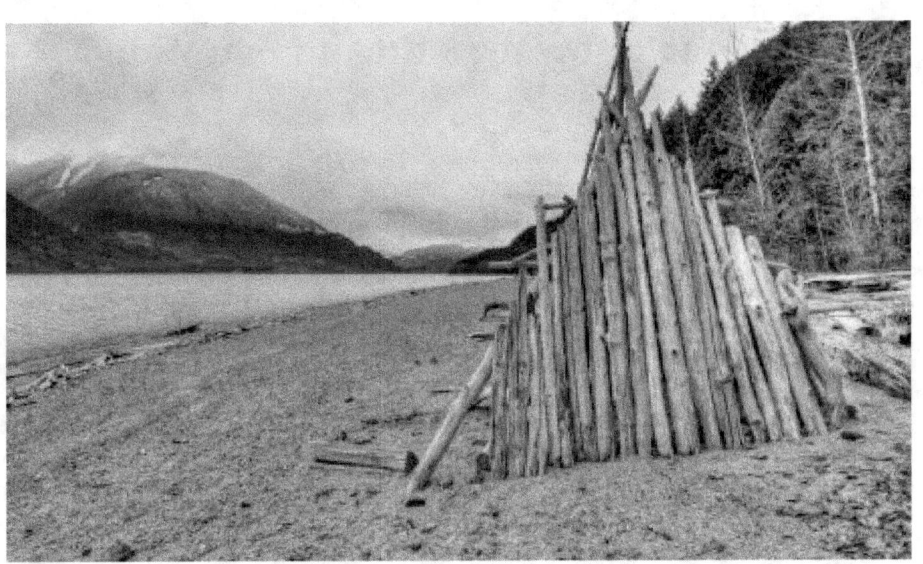

Chapter Four - How to build and maintain a fire

Making, moving, and keeping a fire are one of your number one priorities in any survival situation. Fire provides you with warmth, cooking food, protection, and light. Without fire you may find survival very difficult. As mentioned in the previous pages of this book there are various ways you can create a fire. If you are trying to start one during the day and the sun is out you can do so with a magnifying glass by focusing the suns light through the glass to a pinpoint on some tinder or dried glass. This will only take a few moments and the power of the suns light focused through the glass will create enough smolder to build a fire.

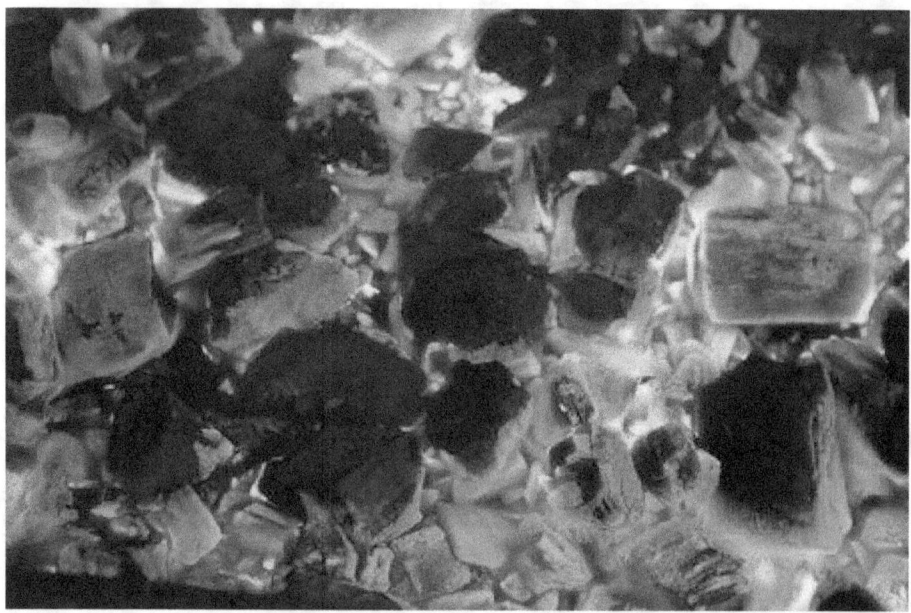

If you are lighting a fire without the sun this is where you waterproof matches will come in handy as well as the lighters you have with you. Find some dry tinder or grass as a starter and add small dry branches and sticks to get the fire a bit bigger. Once the fire is going add a few larger dry pieces of wood to the fire to really get it going well. If you find you have found some wet or even damp wood you can place the wood along the outside of the fire you created to help dry it for future burning. If you find wood and you think it is dry but unsure you can always place it in the fire. If it burns through it is dry, if it burns the outside and the inside along the edges is either steaming or making steam like sounds then the wood is wet and will take much heat to dry it out. You can keep it in the fire however get a long poker stick and keep the wet piece turning this way you dry it all the way.

Now once you have a fire lit it is good to keep it burning as long as possible. So, you must be vigilant and stoke the fire often. Keeping up with adding wood can be tiresome but you are far better with the fire than without it and the work you do to keep it going is worth it in the long run.

If you want to move your fire from one location to another you can do so by many different means. The first and easiest is to use a dry stick and place one end into the fire until it starts to burn. Even if the fire goes out you can still use the hot embers of the stick to start a fire in a different location. To move a fire without a stick you can make a tinder ball which is made up from bark strings, tall dry grasses or even small vines. Place a hot small ember inside the center of the ball and this will provide the ember with enough fuel to be moved from one place to another. Once you have moved the tinder ball to the desired location place the ball into your new fire pit, and begin to blow on the ball it should ignite with little to no effort. Add dry sticks and branches to the tinder and presto, your new fire location has been created.

Chapter Five - Location is Key

Depending on your situation and where you are located will ultimately determine the general outcome of the available items you will have to use for any given survival situation. The biggest key to all of this is knowing what to do and how to act during these kinds of situations. If you are in a tropical setting, you will need more consumable water and high calorie foods. Your shelter will vary in its appearance than the ones we talked about in this book but, your basic needs will be the same to find or build shelter. To maintain your health and to ultimately find a way out of the situation you are surviving in.

If you are in a urban environment you have the ability to use most anything around you as a shelter. Abandoned cars, park pavilions, sheds, the list is endless. Your most difficult scenario may be fending off other would be survivalists in the same situation you are in.

If at all possible in an environment where you will be in close proximity to other people who are not with you or your party, try to find a location that is away from the others and try not to draw attention to yourself. Most people in these types of scenarios do not act with a clear mind and often panic. You do not want to be on that side of the fence if and when this happens.

If you are in the woods or wilderness you will want to find a location near a tree line or near water. You can use the tree line for protection from wind and various types of storms plus, it offers shade from the heat of summer. The water is a great resource for finding wildlife to trap, hunt, or snare. As you need water so do animals in the wild and locating a animal trail by water may help you in staying alive. Also, try and build your shelter near trees on a flat non-swampy clearing. Try to avoid swamp areas all together as these are prone to contamination, stagnation, and plenty of would be insects waiting for a quick lunch.

Remember: Location, location, location.

Chapter Six - Review

1. No matter how you look at it, any survival situation will test your ability and your mind. Always have the proper tools, food, water, and education to help you in any given survival or disaster situation.

2. Be certain to have a plan. Planning the how's and when's will make all the difference in your situation. Make certain you have everything you need or know how to make it.

3. Never assume anything. Survival is never certain and many things can happen that can be for the good or the bad. Be certain you have your bases covered.

4. Never tackle more than you can handle. Take frequent breaks. Remember this is survival and it is very real. Rushing and causing yourself injury in any way should be avoided at all costs.

5. Check and re-check your supply list. Make sure you have everything you need to survive a night or a month.

6. Always bring a basic first aid kit with you for any situation. You never know when you will need it and how much this kit could help save your life.

7. Bring whatever medications you normally take with you. Without these you could put yourself in harm's way.

8. Don't panic. Keep a clear mind and do not allow fear and stress to bring you down.

9. Keep hydrated and fed. These two things are your number one way of surviving. Without food and water you will be putting yourself in a dangerous spot.

10. Failure in survival mode is not an option.

11. Never take risks that have no certain outcome. Everything you do

is survival mode will dictate your situation. Always be safe.

12. Never use fire where you sleep or where it is unsafe.

13. Protect yourself from would be other survivalists in panic mode. Be the leader.

14. When and if the time is right seek help by locating help. Police, Firefighters, the Red Cross. If you see them or find them along the way direct them to your location as there could be others nearby.

In this day and age you never know what is going to happen. However, if disaster strikes, with this book and the information provided you can survive........

About the Author

Born in the Adirondack Mountains of Northern New York State Shannon Rizzotto has been writing since the age of eleven. Since then he has penned three titles of his own as well as countless columns for three newspapers in New York and Vermont. He has been the author of two series online and in print titled, In your backyard, as well as Kids Korner. He is the former editor of BBE Entertainment which conducted online written interviews with bands, models, and photographers the world over. Shannon enjoys writing on survival and medicinal topics and is a certified EMT who enjoys living life in rural upstate New York.

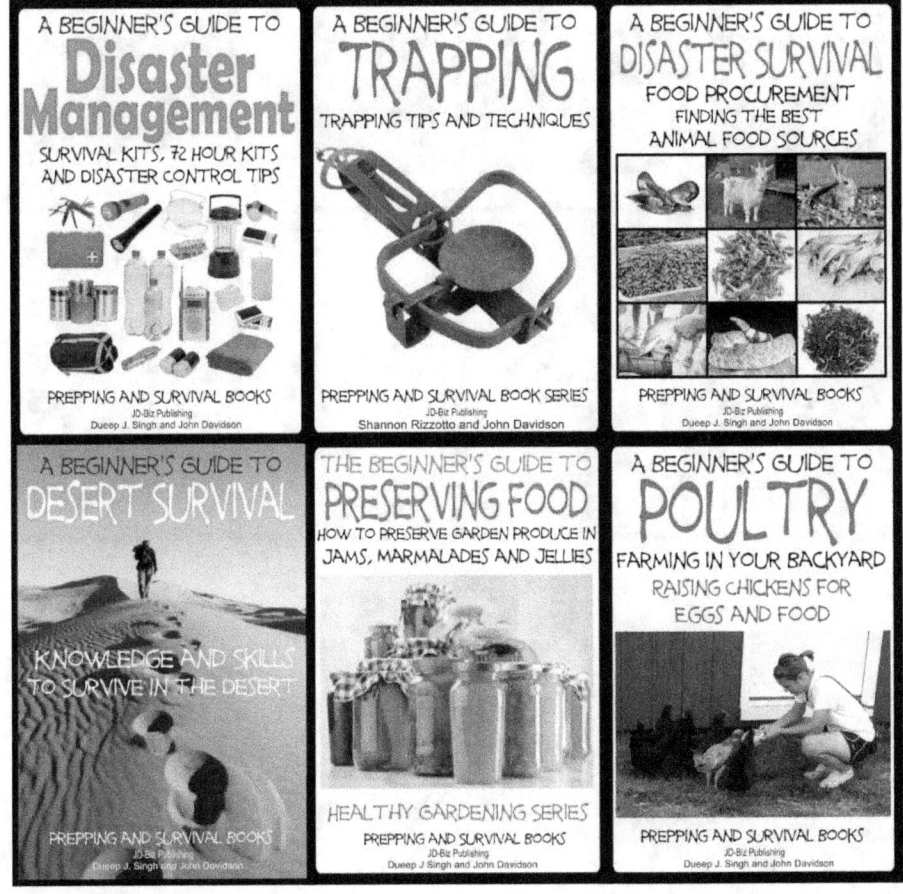

Check out some of the other JD-Biz Publishing books
Gardening Series on Amazon

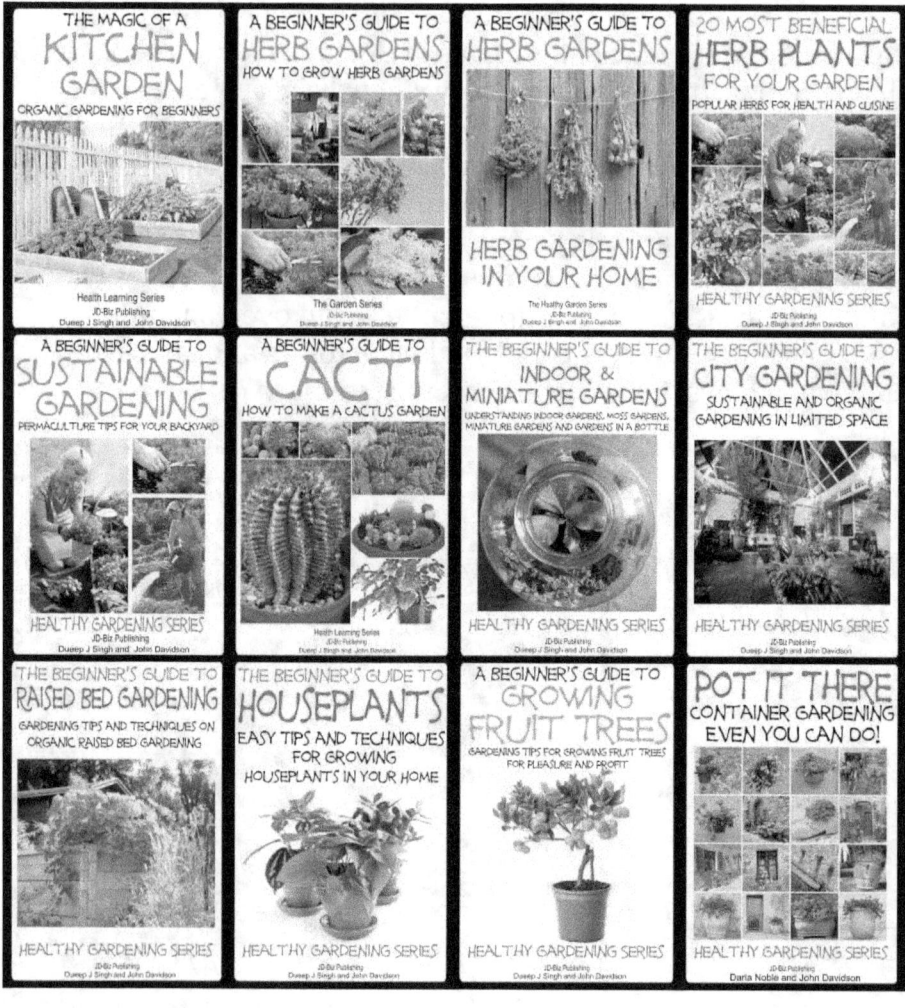

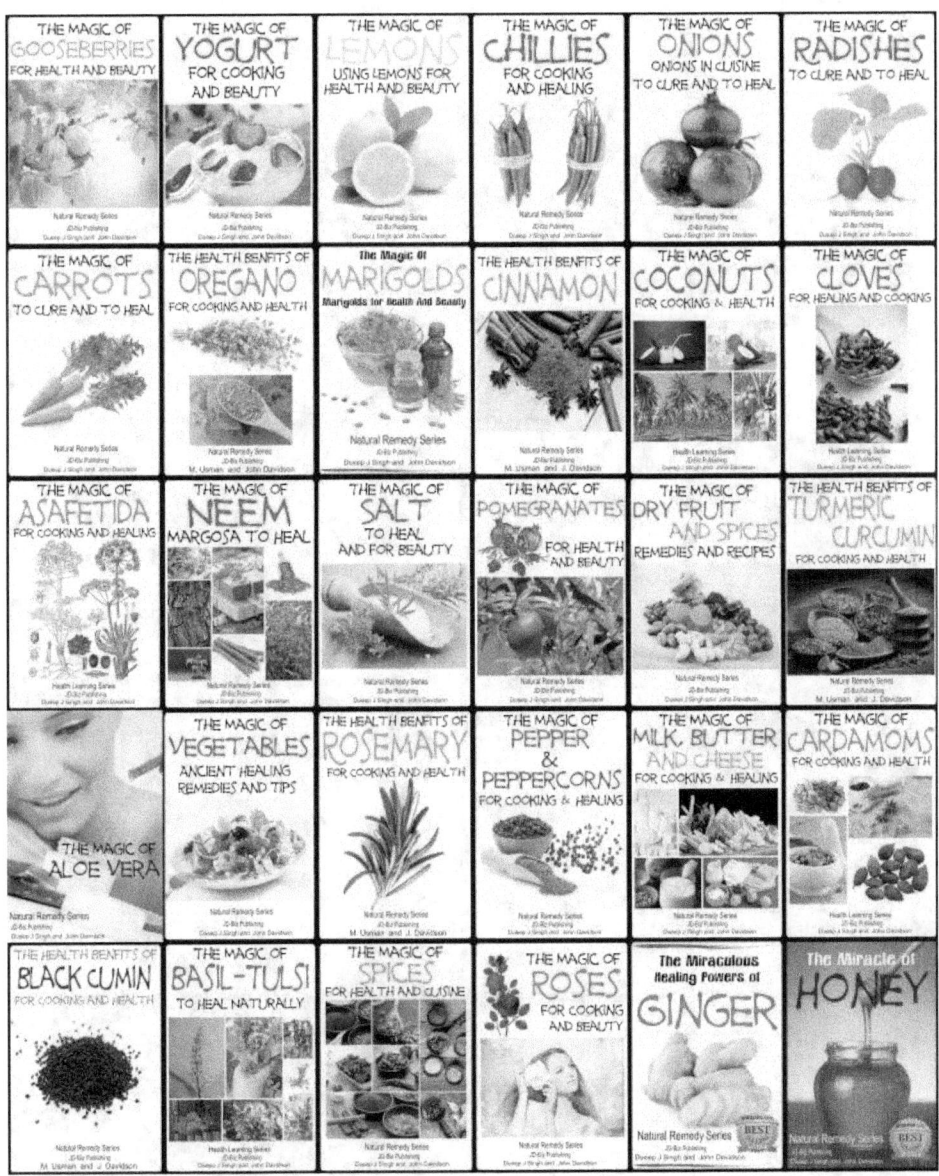

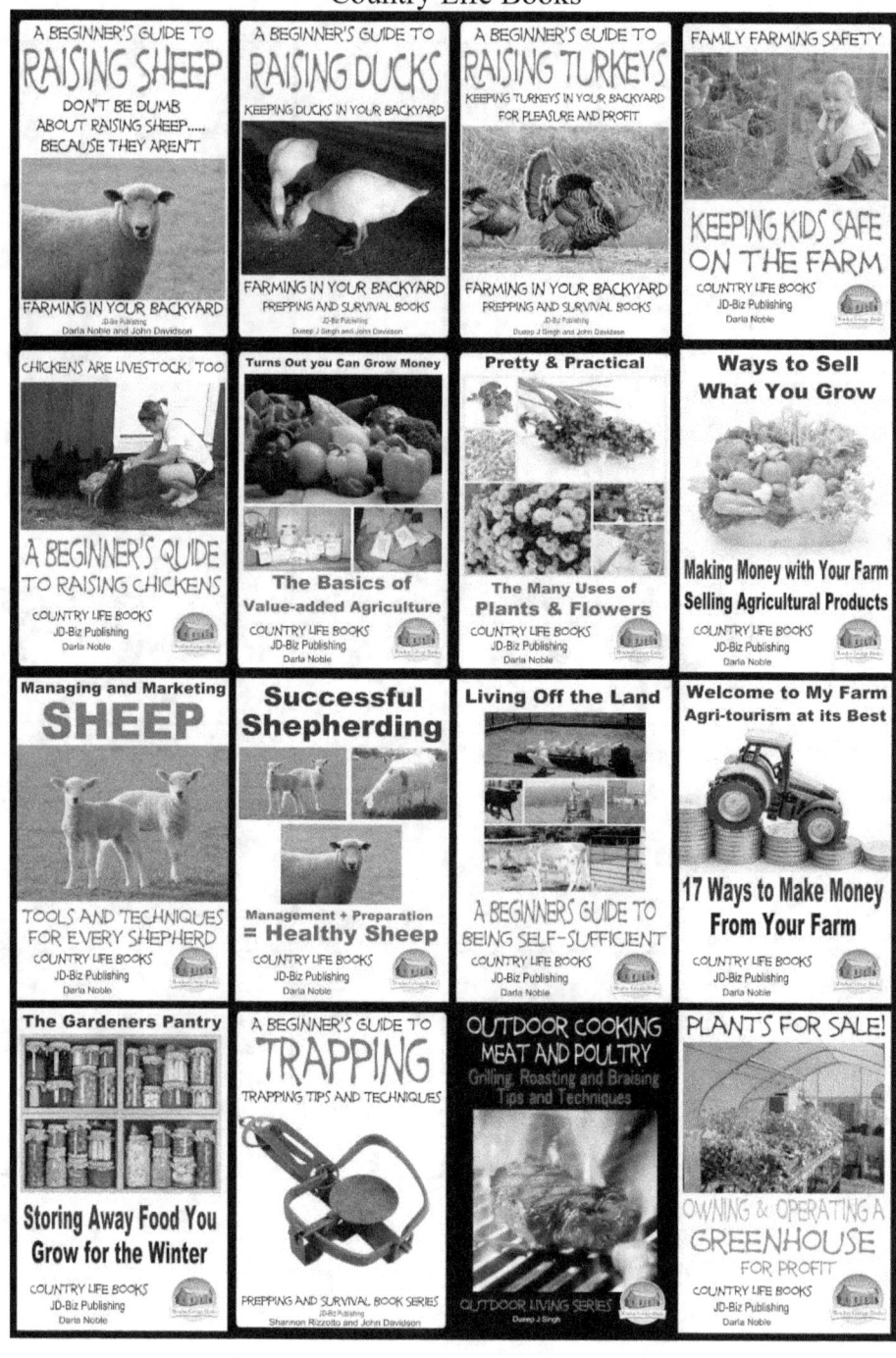

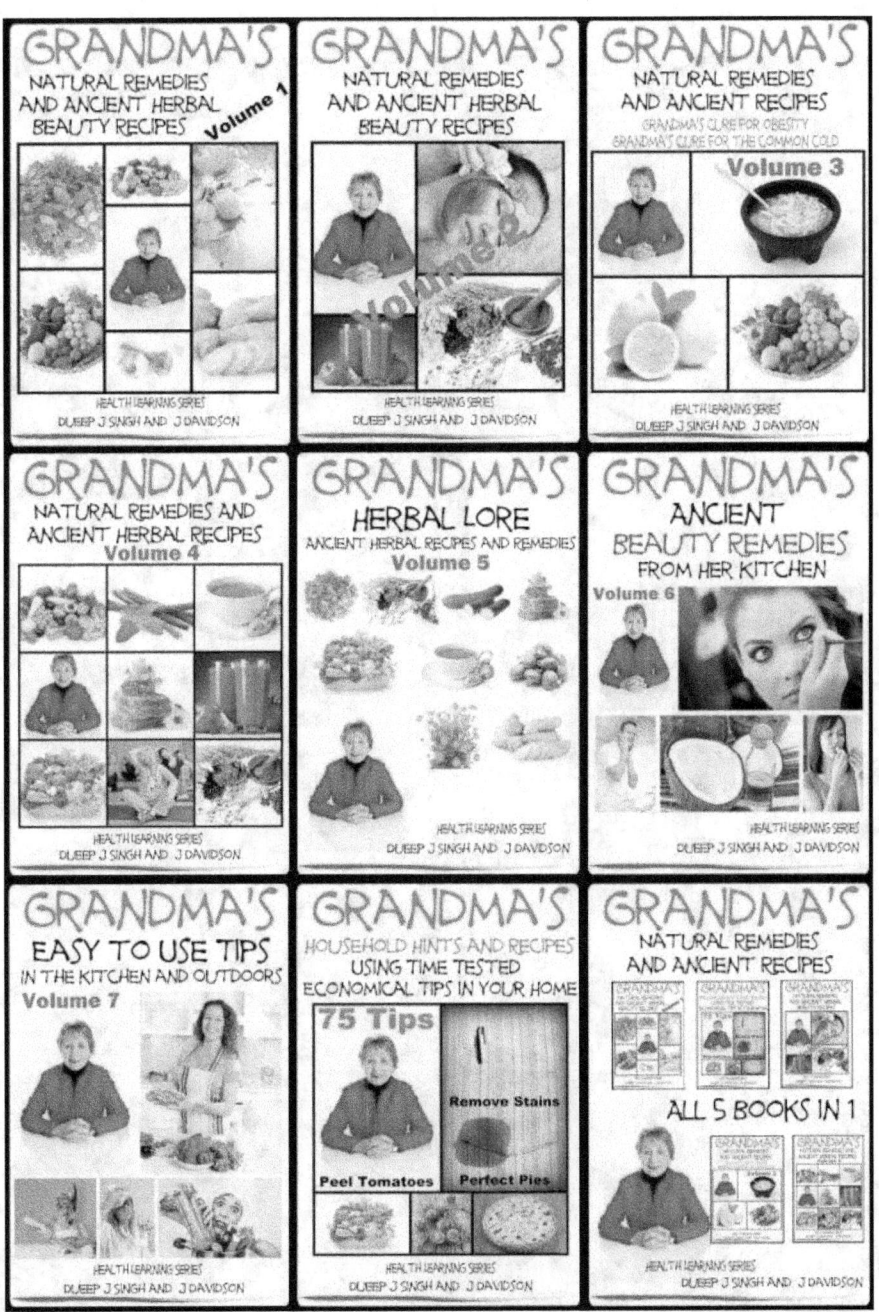

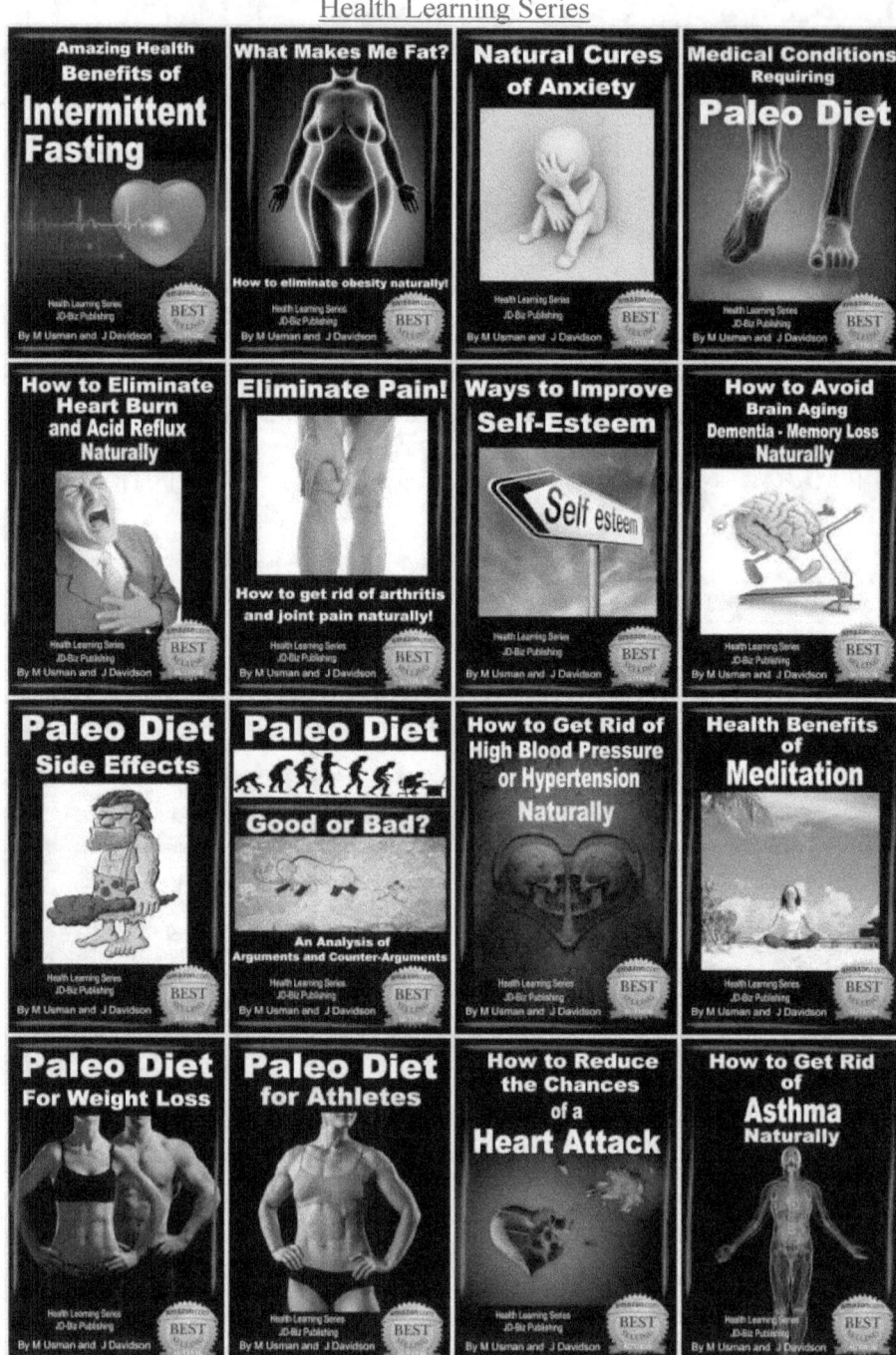

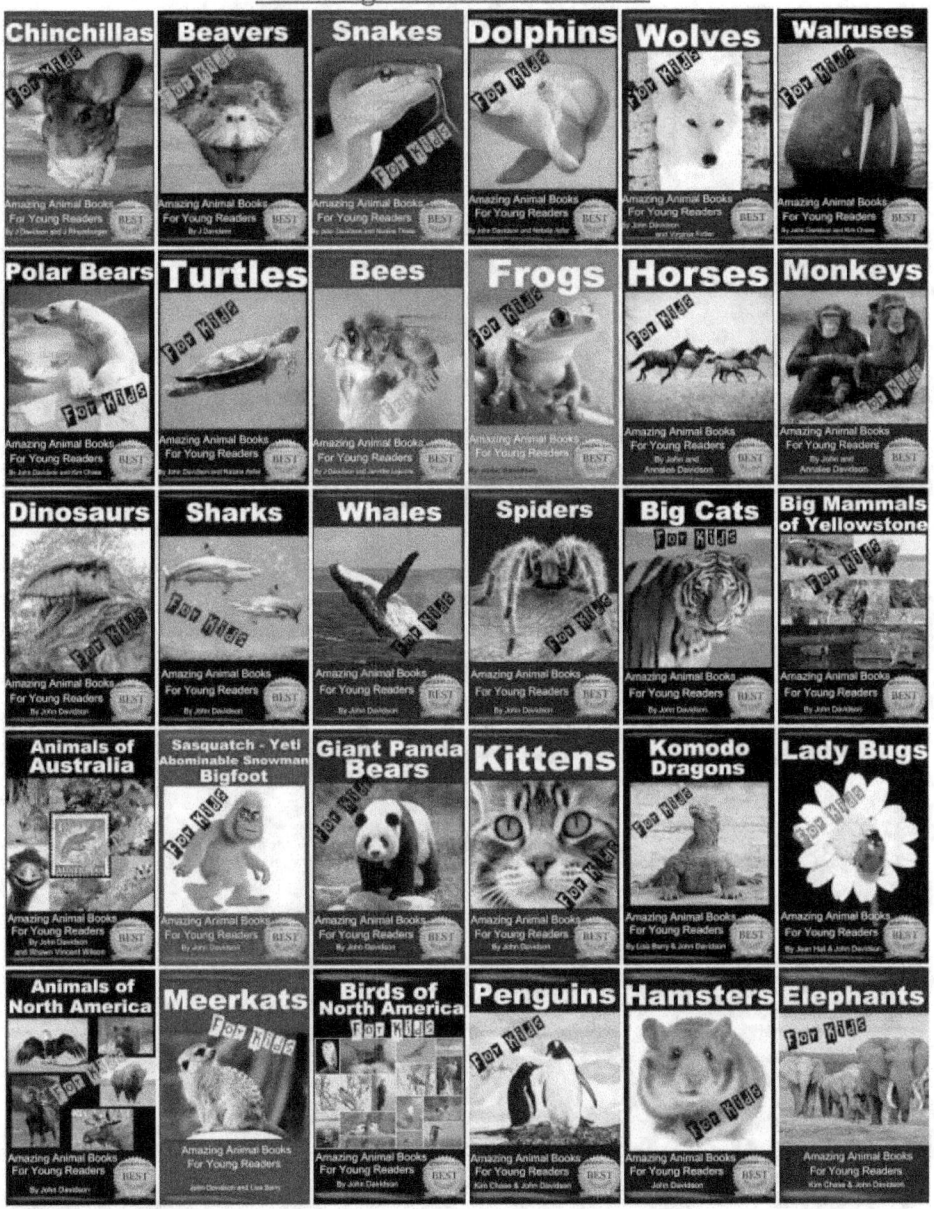

Learn To Draw Series

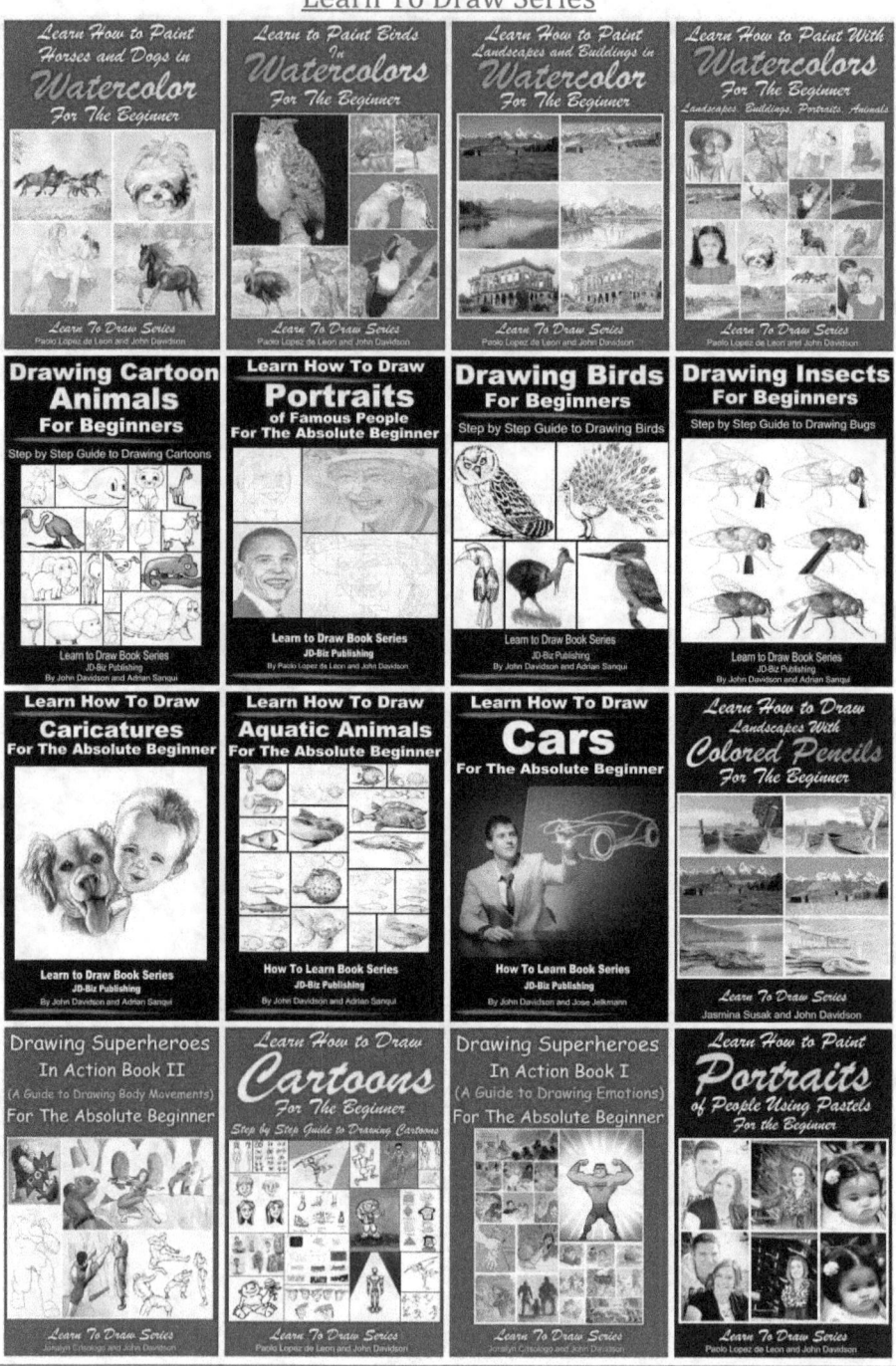

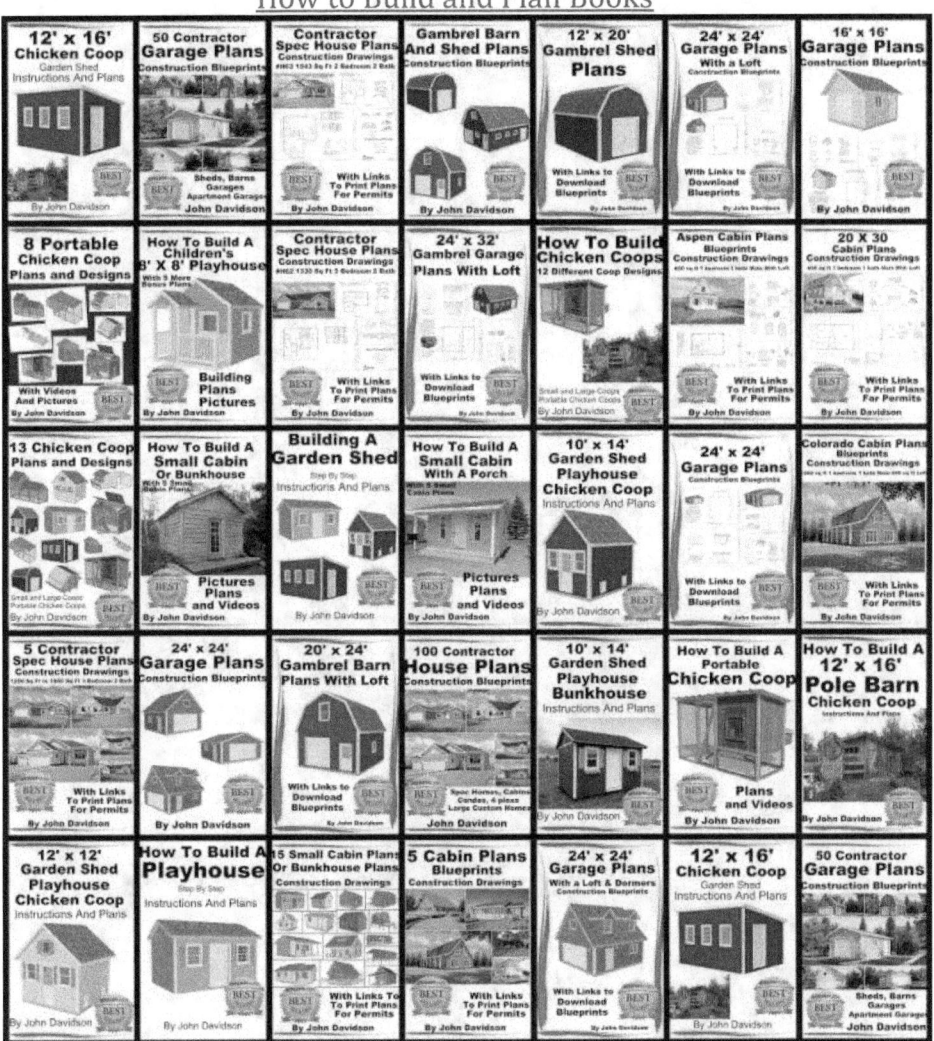

Entrepreneur Book Series

Publisher

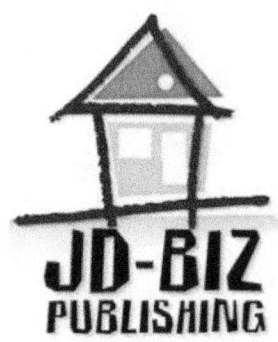

JD-Biz Corp

P O Box 374

Mendon, Utah 84325

http://www.jd-biz.com/

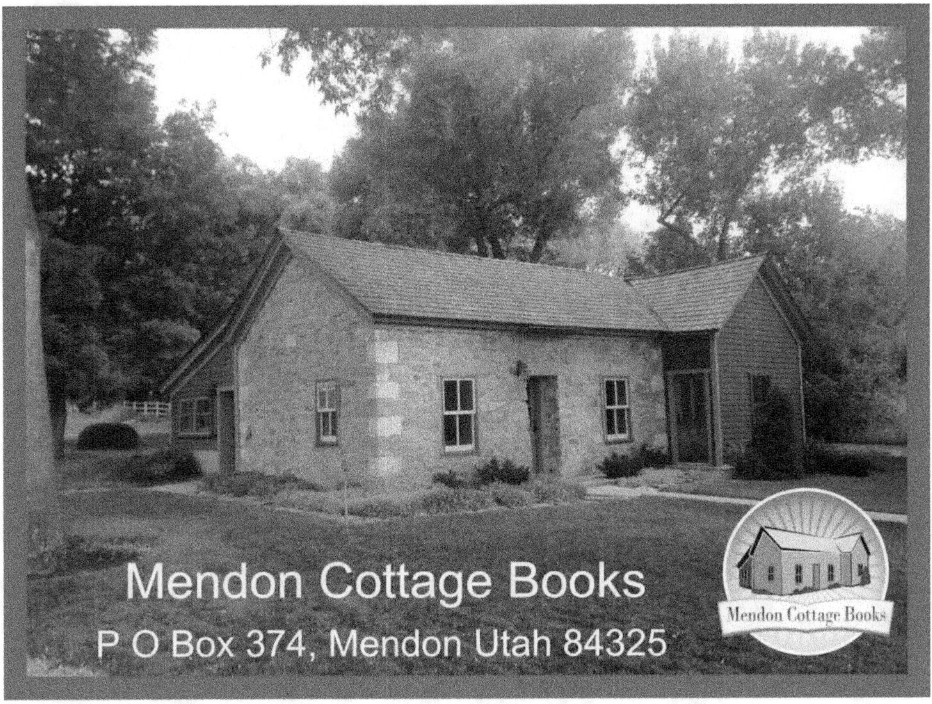

Mendon Cottage Books

P O Box 374, Mendon Utah 84325

Mendon Cottage Books